50 MATHEMATICAL PUZZLES AND PROBLEMS

ORANGE COLLECTION

From the International Championship of Mathematics
Fédération Française des Jeux Mathématiques

Gilles Cohen, Editor
Éditions POLE

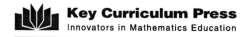

Key Curriculum Press
Innovators in Mathematics Education

Éditions POLE

Coordinator: Michel Criton

Translator: Jean-Christophe Novelli

Editor: Gilles Cohen

Reading and Editing Committee: Julien Cassaigne, Francis Gutmacher, Jon Millington, Bernard Novelli, Jean-Christophe Novelli, Lucien Pianaro

Problem Authors: Jean-Claude Bartier, Gilles Cohen, Gérard Crézé, Michel Criton, Nicolas Didrit, Gilles Flament, Robert Gérardy, Francis Gutmacher, Patrice Lucas, Bernard Novelli, Zbigniew Romanowicz, Dominique Souder

Key Curriculum Press

Project Administrator: Heather Dever

Editorial Assistant: Kyle Bridget Loftus

Mathematics and Translation Reviewer: Dudley Brooks

Production Editor: Jennifer Strada

Copy Editor: Margaret Moore

Production Director: Diana Jean Parks

Production Coordinator: Laurel Roth Patton

Compositor: Laurel Roth Patton

Cover Designer: Caroline Ayres

Prepress and Printer: Malloy Lithographing, Inc.

Executive Editor: Casey FitzSimons

Publisher: Steven Rasmussen

Key Curriculum Press, 1150 65th Street, Emeryville, CA 94608, 510-595-7000
editorial@keypress.com
http://www.keypress.com

Éditions POLE, 31 Avenue des Gobelins, 75013 Paris, France

Printed in the United States of America
10 9 8 7 6 5 4 3
ISBN 978-1-55953-499-4

❖ PREFACE ❖

The International Championship of Mathematics and Logic has been held in France by the FFJM (Fédération Française des Jeux Mathématiques) for more than ten years. Writers for these championships have generated over a thousand original puzzles, which are regularly gathered and published in French by Éditions POLE. Key Curriculum Press is pleased to be able to offer a selection of these problems, translated into English.

The problems are organized by difficulty in three collections: the *Green Collection* (grades 6 through 12), the *Orange Collection* (grades 9 through 12), and the *Red Collection* (grade 9 through college level). Full solutions are provided in each book.

We hope you will enjoy these problems. We invite you to participate with the 150,000 other contestants in the International Championship of Mathematics and Logic, which is held once a year in France. For more information, please write to:

FFJM, 1 Avenue Foch, 94700 Maison-Alfort, France

As you work these problems, keep in mind the essential goals of the championship: to apply reasoning more than knowledge, and to find not only one but all of the solutions to a problem.

Éditions POLE
Key Curriculum Press

❖ CONTENTS ❖

Chapter 4 ❖ Equations, Inequalities, and Systems

Chapter 5 ❖ Algorithms

Chapter 6 ❖ Logical Questions

CHAPTER I

Symmetry

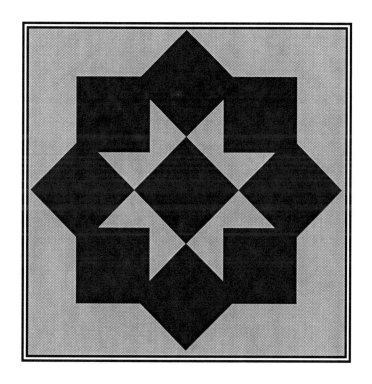

1 ❖ The Eight Pieces

Cut this hexagon into eight pieces of the same size and shape (rotated or reflected).

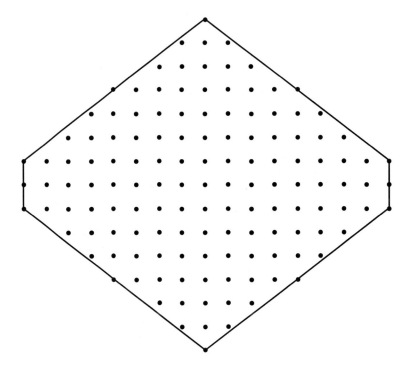

2 ❖ The Four Strings

Four pieces of string of lengths 3 meters, 5 meters, 11 meters, and 13 meters are tied in a single knot. You pull the four strings so that their free ends form the vertices of a quadrilateral.

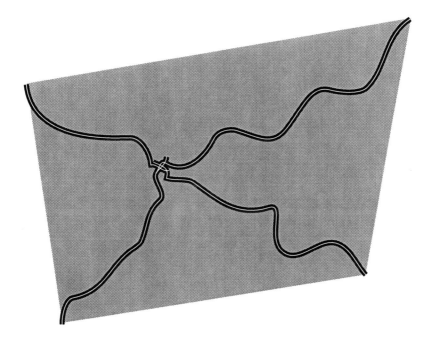

❖ Find the maximum possible area of this quadrilateral.

Give your answer in square meters, rounded to the nearest integer.

Note: You can ignore the length of string used to tie the knot.

3 ❖ The Cut Square

A straight line cuts the perimeter of this square into two parts, whose lengths are 35 centimeters and 21 centimeters. This line cuts one side of the square into two segments of lengths 1 centimeter and 13 centimeters and another side into two segments of lengths 6 centimeters and 8 centimeters.

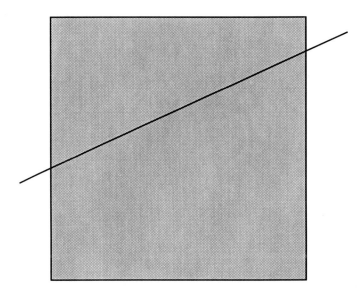

❖ What is the area of the smaller part of the square?

Give the answer(s) in square centimeters.

4 ❖ Rose's Scarf

This scarf cost a lot! Its shape is a right triangle in which the square *ROSE* is inscribed.

The scarf's price in French Francs is the same as the area of *ROSE* in square centimeters. We know only that $AE = 12$ centimeters and $SI = 27$ centimeters.

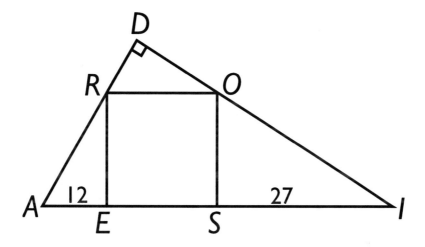

❖ How much did the scarf cost?

5 ❖ Crosses on a Checkerboard

You have a 5 × 7 checkerboard and an unlimited number of "cards," each of which consists of five squares assembled to form a cross.

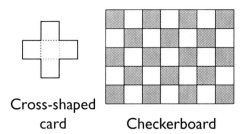

Cross-shaped card   Checkerboard

Place the cards one by one on the checkerboard so that at least one square of each card coincides with a square on the checkerboard.

The game is over when all the squares of the checkerboard are covered.

❖ What is the minimum number of cards you would use, if you played your best?

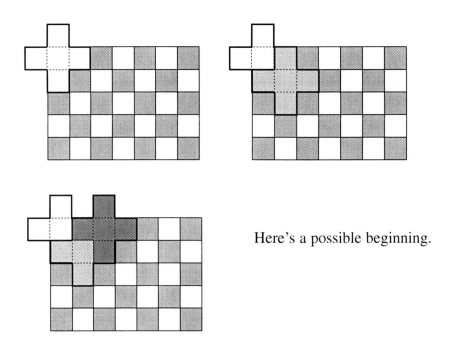

Here's a possible beginning.

6 ✧ Leo's Transmissions

Leo is a garage mechanic as efficient as he is shrewd. His sign is a
3 × 20 rectangle containing the shapes of the 12 pentominoes. Among
those, he has used red ink to color the initials of his garage and a small car.

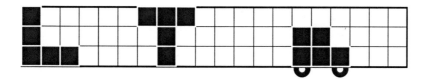

❖ Fill in the rectangle with the 9 remaining pentominoes, shown below.

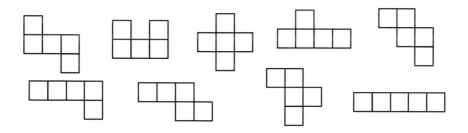

Note: You can rotate or turn over any pentomino as necessary.

7 ❖ Four Colors for a Coloring

You have four colors at your disposal: black, blue (**B**), white, and red (**R**).

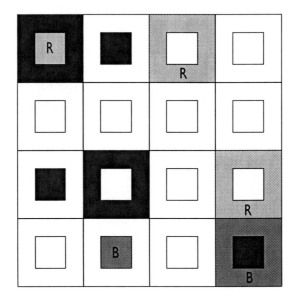

❖ Fill in the picture according to these rules:

- Each square is two-colored (the center and the border are different colors).
- In each row of four squares (horizontal, vertical, or diagonal), all the centers have different colors and all the borders have different colors.

Note: None of the white centers or borders are indicated yet. Anything that appears white here may in fact be any color.

8 ❖ The Three-Colored Knights

Once upon a time, a handsome knight with a three-colored helmet (see below) came to the farthest bounds of our country. To the people who asked him where he came from, he answered:

"My country is divided into counties. In each county, all the knights wear helmets like mine. The upper part (surrounded by a bold line) of all the helmets of my country is identically colored. (Note: The three colors are represented by black, white, and gray.) The lower part (not colored in the picture) differs from county to county. All helmet coloring abides by these rules:

- Each color is used three times.
- Two identical colors are never adjacent.

"Finally, you need to know that all possible color combinations are used."

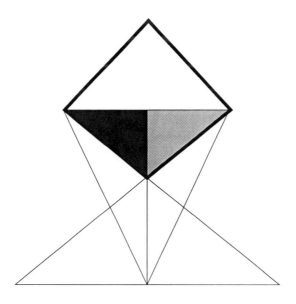

❖ How many counties are there in the knight's country?

---

9 ❖ The Four-Color Process

To test new products, Mr. Lechat builds an experimental model. He associates a color with each of his four products, and he creates a 4 × 4 × 4 cube so that each row of four small cubes (except diagonals) contains the four colors, white, green, black, and violet.

He has just finished building his cube, but he didn't have time to finish the coloring. The V indicates a violet face and the G a green face.

You know that there is a white cube below the violet cube in the left rear corner of the top layer.

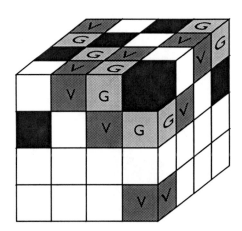

❖ What are the colors of the cubes in the first two layers, starting from the bottom?

Use W, G, B, and V for white, green, black, and violet.

CHAPTER 2

Divisions and Fractions

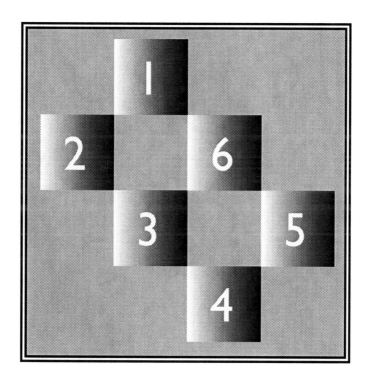

10 ❖ Surrounding 55

Granddad Joss would like you to fill in the eight circles around 55 with different numbers less than 100 so that the product of any three numbers in a line always equals 1,980.

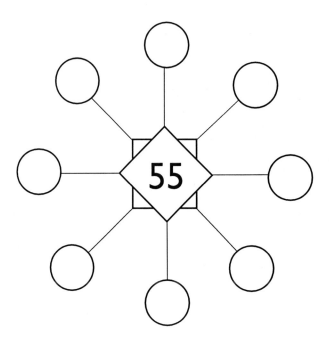

❖ What is the sum of the eight numbers surrounding 55?

11 ❖ Matthew and Multiples

"**Y**ou never know what my grandpa Joss is going to make up next!" says Matthew to his friend Matilda. "He gave me this array to fill with twelve numbers; each has to satisfy the "yes" and "no" of its row and also the conditions of the columns a and b!"

	The nearest number to 95 ↓	Divisible by						The nearest number to 196 ↓
a		**2**	**3**	**4**	**5**	**7**	**9**	**b**
		yes	yes	yes	no	no	yes	
		no	no	no	yes	yes	no	
		yes	yes	no	no	yes	no	
		no	no	no	no	no	no	
		yes	yes	yes	yes	no	no	
		yes	no	no	yes	yes	no	

"My grandpa is quite a trickster. He promised me that if everything was right, I would receive for my birthday—that is tomorrow—an amount of money (in French Francs) equal to the sum of the twelve numbers!"

"I see. So, you're asking me to help you, right? OK, we'll make it fifty-fifty," says Matilda.

❖ Matthew and Matilda found all the numbers. How many French Francs did Matilda earn?

12 ❖ Truncadivisible

If you take the number 24 and remove its units digit (4), 2 remains, and 24 is divisible by 2. Such a number, which happens to be divisible by itself truncated by its units digit, is called a "truncadivisible" number.

❖ How many "truncadivisible" numbers less than 1,995 are there?

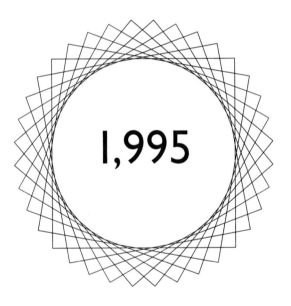

13 ❖ The Karr Brothers

The well-known Karr brothers, who live in the small village of Mazoff, are more than two but fewer than ten.

They are all sheep ranchers, and their herds are their only wealth. The numbers of animals in their herds are consecutive numbers. The total number of sheep is 1,995.

❖ How many sheep does the least wealthy Karr brother have?

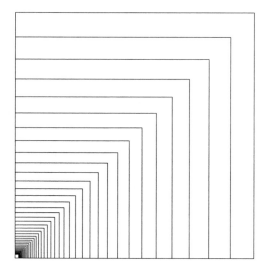

14 ❖ Little House on the Prairie

It takes my dad 6 hours to hoe our garden. When Grandpa Joss comes to visit us, it takes him 10 hours to do the same amount of work. Today, they have decided to work together.

❖ How long will it take Dad and Grandpa to hoe the whole garden?

Give the answer in minutes.

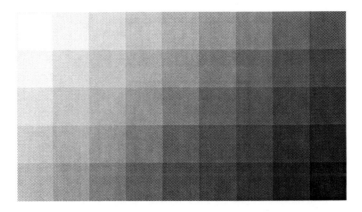

15 ❖ Of Dice and Decimals

Lisa's father gave her one red die and one green die. She uses them to make up fractions, with the numerator given by the green die and the denominator given by the red die.

Some of these fractions are terminating decimals (for example, you get 0.5 with a 3 on the green die and a 6 on the red die, since 3/6 = 0.5) and some are not (for example, you get 0.66666 . . . , with a green 2 and a red 3, and the division never ends).

❖ How many different terminating decimal results can Lisa get with these two dice?

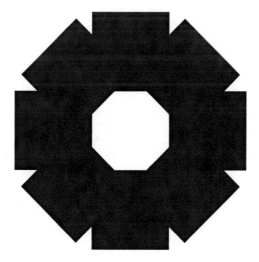

16 ❖ Stacking Fractions

If you "stack" the numbers 1, 2, and 3 in a fraction, you can get two different results: 1/6 and 3/2, depending on which division you do first:

$$\frac{\frac{1}{2}}{3} = \frac{1}{6} \quad \text{and} \quad \frac{1}{\frac{2}{3}} = \frac{3}{2}$$

❖ How many different results can you get by "stacking" into a complex fraction the numbers 1, 2, 3, 4, 5, 6, 7, and 8, in that order?

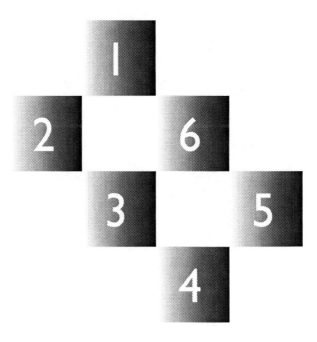

CHAPTER 3

Computations Galore

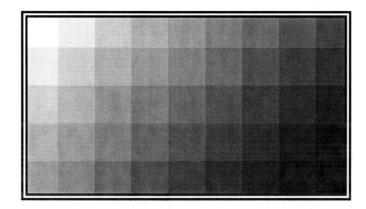

17 ❖ Palindrome

In the movie *Tandem,* by Patrice Leconte, the actor Jean Rochefort looks at his car's odometer and, reading 83238, explains that it is a palindrome. It is the same read from left to right and from right to left. Then he remarks that the next palindrome will be 83338.

❖ What will be the seventh palindrome after 83338?

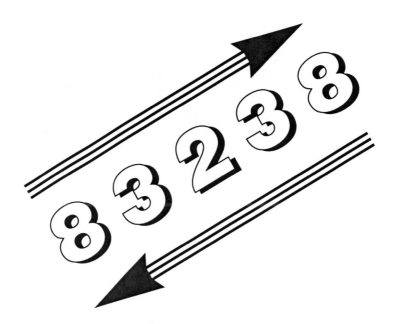

18 ❖ The Quasi-Perfect Years

The year 1996 was quasi-perfect because one of the numbers obtained by deleting a single digit is a perfect square. Specifically, deleting a 9 gives 196, the square of 14.

❖ Before 1996, how many quasi-perfect years were there in the 1900s?

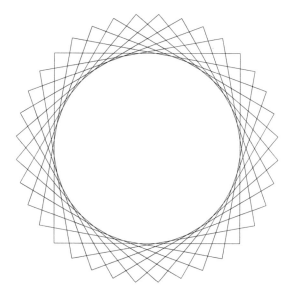

19 ❖ Heads or Tails?

Lira spends all her time inventing games with her collection of coins. This time, she has set out four coins, heads up. In the first move, she turns over the first coin. In the second move, she turns over the first two coins; in the third move, she turns over the first three coins; the fourth move, the first four coins. On the fifth move, she starts all over again, turning over the first coin, and so on.

❖ What are the sides of the four coins after 1,995 moves?

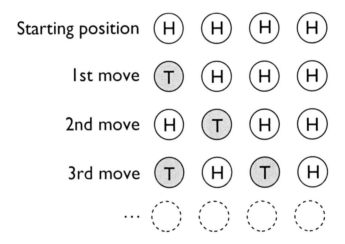

50 Mathematical Puzzles and Problems ◆ *Orange Collection*
©2001 Key Curriculum Press

20 ❖ Sommersby

Sommersby is conducting a training exercise with his toy soldiers. He forms two teams: On the left side, he puts his 95 orange soldiers (his favorite); on the right side, he puts 51 green and 15 blue soldiers. At the end of each round, 2 green soldiers, 1 blue soldier, and 1 orange soldier are eliminated. To balance the game, Sommersby decides that, between rounds, the green-and-blue team will get as many new green soldiers as there are blue soldiers left.

❖ How many rounds will be necessary to entirely eliminate one of the two teams? Which team will win, and how many soldiers will be left?

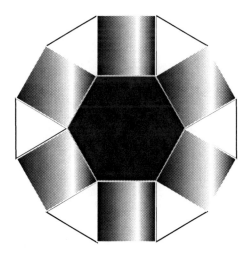

21 ❖ The Magic Wheel

The circles in the wheel shown below contain the numbers from 1 to 7. This wheel is "magic"; that is, the sum of three numbers in a row is constant.

❖ What is the number in the center of the wheel?

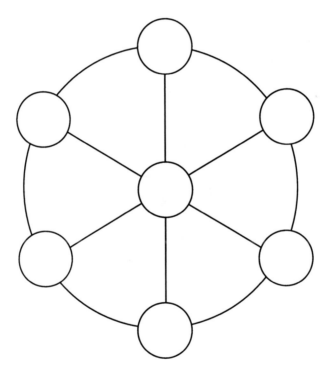

22 ❖ Missing Numbers

Romeo and Juliet are two 10-year-old students. Their teacher gave them a multiplication table with missing numbers to fill in (e.g., $8 \times 5 = 40$).

Romeo and Juliet compare their results: They agree about A, but they disagree about B.

×			5	
		12		6
		24		A
8			40	
	63	B		

❖ Knowing that all factors (such as 5 and 8) are greater than 1 and smaller than 10, find all the possible values of B.

23 ❖ The Raffle

Alice, Bob, Chris, David, and Elizabeth participate in a raffle. Inside a hat are cards numbered from 1 to 12, each number corresponding to a winning prize. Each participant picks two cards but, to make a game of it, they give only the sum of their cards: Alice declares 11, Bob 4, Chris 16, David 7, and Elizabeth 19.

❖ Find the smaller number picked by each participant.

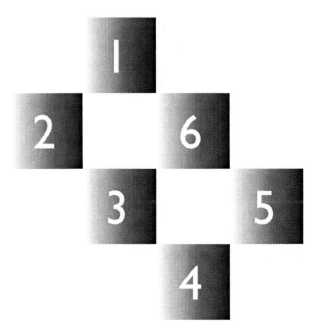

24 ❖ The Nine Numbers

You write the numbers from 1 to 81 in a 9 × 9 square, as shown in the table (filling the successive rows, from left to right, then from right to left, then from left to right, and so on). You then choose nine numbers in this square so that no two of them belong to the same row or the same column.

❖ What is the maximum possible value of the sum of these nine numbers?

1	2	3	4	5	6	7	8	9
18	17	16	15	14	13	12	11	10
19	...							
						...	80	81

25 ❖ Ninety-nine

1 2 3 4 5 6 7 8 9

In this sequence of the digits from 1 to 9, you can get many different numbers by inserting plus signs. For instance:

$$1234 + 567 + 89 = 1{,}890$$
$$1 + 23 + 4 + 56 + 7 + 89 = 180$$

❖ Insert plus signs in this sequence of digits to get 99.

CHAPTER 4

Equations, Inequalities, and Systems

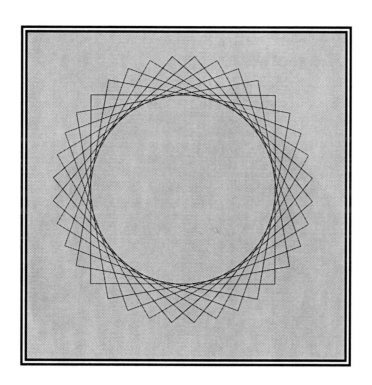

26 ❖ The Compact Disk

The last CD of the MatheMatics costs a whole number of French Francs. Although his piggy bank is not empty, Matthew cannot buy it since he is 47 French Francs short. The same goes for Matilda; she is 2 French Francs short. Matilda and Matthew decide to pool their money to buy the CD. Alas, they still don't have enough to buy it.

❖ What is the price of the MatheMatics CD?

27❖Full House

Jenny says: "I'm the sixth child in my family, and I have at least as many brothers as I have sisters." Her brother Jim adds, "I have at least twice as many sisters as brothers."

❖ How many girls and boys are in Jenny and Jim's family?

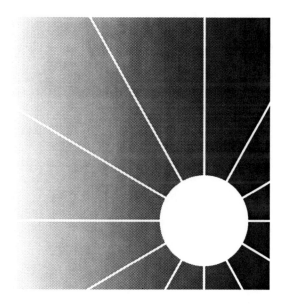

28 ❖ Where's He From?

P̲hil's car is registered in a region of France. His license plate number is shown below. The last two digits, represented by the two question marks, are the region's number. The sum of these digits is equal to the difference between 94 and this number.

❖ What is the region's number?

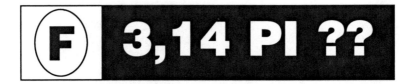

29 ❖ Encyclonumberist

Dennis loves his encyclopedia. Today, he opens it at random. The numbers on the two pages he is looking at are three-digit numbers, the one on the left page being, as usual, even. Writing these two numbers requires only three different digits, which are consecutive. One of these digits was used three times, another twice, and the last digit once. The sum of these six digits is 25.

❖ What is the number on the left page?

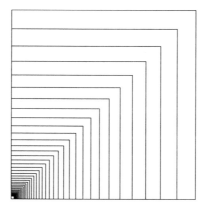

30 ❖ Maggie's Birth Month

Start with Maggie's birth month. Multiply it by 4. Add to this product the difference between 12 and her birth month. Subtract from this result twice the sum of 5 and her birth month.

❖ If you end up with 10, what must Maggie's birth month be?

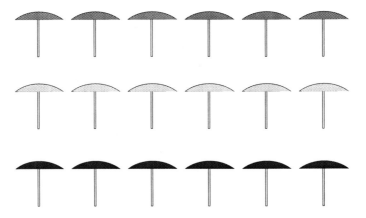

31 ❖ An Interesting Property

Mr. Gideon owns a large piece of land. The exact shape of his land is shown below. All sides of the property are the same length. As well as its shape, it has another curious property: If you compute its perimeter in kilometers and its area in square kilometers, the results are the same!

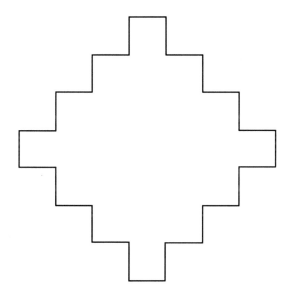

❖ What is the perimeter of Mr. Gideon's property in meters?

32 ❖ Numerical Polygons

Diana Jones and her twin brother, Kevin, are at the end of a corridor inside the pyramid of Keplus Keminus. The heavy door in front of them will move only if they press the right stones on a great wall.

The instructions state that each stone contains an "invisible" number. Each number is the result of performing the indicated operation on the number in the previous stone, when following the polygonal paths. To open the door, the twins have to press three stones of identical value.

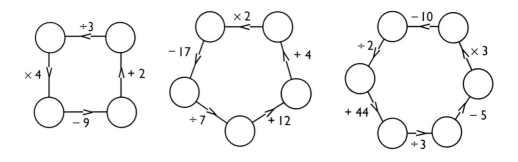

❖ Find one of the possible values.

33 ❖ The Lucky Year

The lucky year was a year after 1000 and before 2000. If you take the lucky year's first two digits and its last two, you obtain 2 two-digit numbers. The lucky part is that twice the product of these numbers is equal to the lucky-year number.

❖ What was this lucky year?

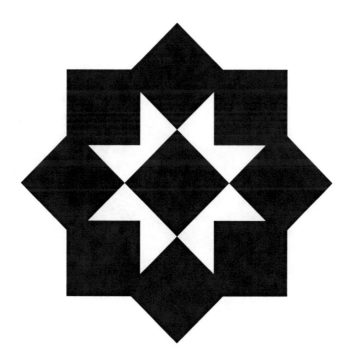

34 ❖ Diana Jones's Suitcase

Diana Jones comes back from Africa with some live animals.

"Anything to declare?" asks the customs officer at the airport.

"Animals, with a total of 7 heads and 28 legs," Diana answers mischievously.

"Open your case!"

The customs officer hurries away when he sees that the suitcase is full of snakes, spiders, and crabs.

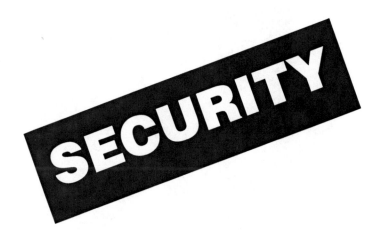

❖ How many of each animal does Diana have in her suitcase?

Reminder: Crabs have ten legs, spiders have eight, and snakes have none. As for the heads . . .

---

35 ❖ The Great Current

Floating down a river, it takes a barge 2 hours to cover 60 kilometers. Going back up the river, it takes the barge 3 hours.

❖ What is the speed of the current, assuming that it is constant?

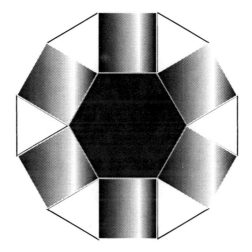

36 ❖ The Three Couples

Three couples, Alice and Dan, Betty and Earl, and Carolyn and Frank, go to the movies. All together, their ages add up to 137 years. Betty's and Earl's ages add up to 47 years. Alice is the oldest woman; she is 4 years older than the youngest woman. Each man is 5 years older than his wife.

❖ How old is each man?

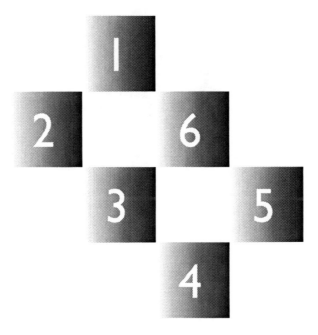

CHAPTER 5

Algorithms

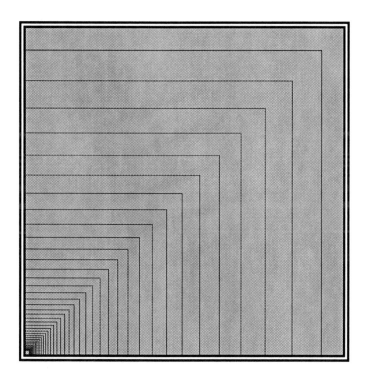

37 ❖ The V.H.L.

The Very High Ladder has an infinite number of equally spaced rungs. Milo goes up the ladder, 13 rungs at a time. After the first jump (of 13 rungs), Milo takes a break during which he goes down one rung. After the second jump, he is even more tired and so he goes down two rungs. Getting more and more exhausted, after the third jump, he goes down three rungs, and so on.

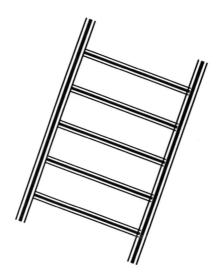

❖ After how many jumps will Milo reach the floor?

Answer 0 if you think that he will never reach the floor.

38 ❖ Lucy's Laces

Lucy always has a pair of laces in her pocket. Each afternoon, before leaving school, she makes a balance sheet of the day's grades. For all the grades greater than or equal to 10 (she always begins with these), she ties a double knot in her laces (see the diagram), two double knots always being separated by a small space. For all the grades smaller than 10, she unties a single knot (if there is any knot left to untie).

But, if at the end of this operation a single knot remains at the end of the laces, it disappears on her way back home.

On Monday morning, both laces were untied. Here are her grades for the week:

Monday: 11, 14
Tuesday: 8, 18, 13
Thursday: 16, 7, 14
Friday: 6, 9, 7

❖ On Friday night, how many knots remained in Lucy's laces? (Each double knot counts as two knots.)

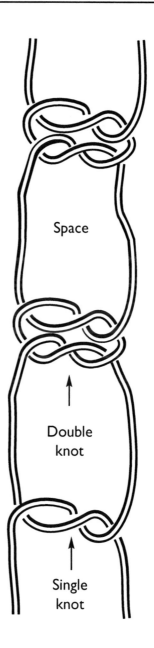

Space

Double knot

Single knot

39 ❖ Sum Up the Neighbors

Chris, who is an excellent table-tennis player, found an original way of showing the score of his often unfortunate opponents.

Six ping-pong balls numbered 1 to 6 (but not in that order) are permanently arranged in a circle. At the end of each round, Chris reads out a series of numbers written on adjacent balls, whose values add up to his opponent's score.

In ping-pong, any score from 1 to 21 is possible; he may need to read from one to six adjacent balls.

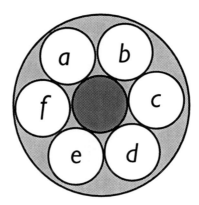

❖ If $a = 1$, $b < f$, and two consecutive numbers are never written on adjacent balls, find the numbers written on the balls.

40 ❖ Doubly True

In this cryptarithm, as in every cryptarithm, different letters always represent diffe-
rent digits, and different digits are always represented by different letters.
Also, no number begins with a 0. The addition below reads, once translated:
SIX + FIVE = ELEVEN.

$$
\begin{array}{r}
\text{S I X} \\
+ \text{ C I N Q} \\
\hline
\text{O N Z E}
\end{array}
$$

❖ Find the smallest and the greatest possible values of ONZE.

41 ❖ Taking Photos

Nine friends who had lost sight of each other for a long time meet at a party and decide to take photos. They want their picture-taking to meet these conditions:

- Each photo must show exactly three of them.
- Each participant will choose only photos in which he doesn't appear, but he must have pictures of all his friends.

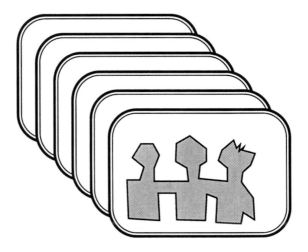

❖ What is the minimum number of photos that enables the nine friends to meet these conditions?

Note: Each photo can be developed as many times as necessary.

42 ❖ Drawing Straws

Five players in a game, Allen, Bob, Chris, Dan, and Edward, are drawing straws. Before each round, each player bets a sum of money and puts it in front of him. Before the first round, Allen bets more than Bob, who bets more than Chris, who bets more than Dan, who bets more than Edward. In each round, the loser has to pay each other player the amount that other player has in front of him, taking the money out of his own (the loser's) pile. If the loser doesn't have enough, he forfeits all his money.

After five rounds, none of the five players has quit the game yet. Each has lost exactly once and has 32 French Francs in front of him.

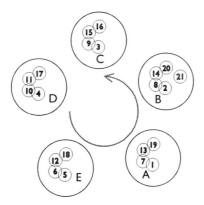

❖ What was the initial bet of each player, from Allen to Edward, at the beginning of the game?

43 ❖ The Willows

At the edge of a pond, there are five marvelous willows in whose branches are no more than 30 sparrows.

First, a sparrow moved from the first willow to the second. Next, two sparrows moved from the second willow to the third, then three sparrows from the third willow to the fourth, four sparrows from the fourth willow to the fifth, and finally, five sparrows from the fifth willow to the first. At the end of this dance, all willows have the same number of sparrows.

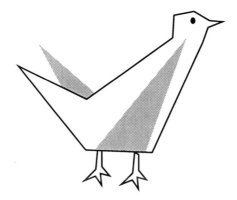

❖ Give the number of sparrows on each willow before their dance.

Logical Questions

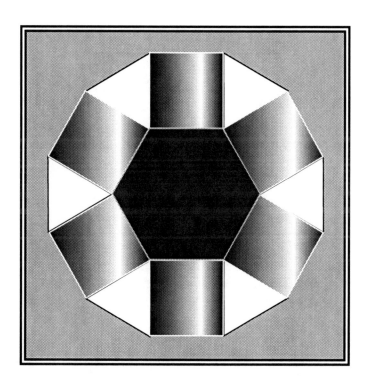

44 ❖ Troy Moves

Some archaeologists recently discovered a very old game that was in use in the ancient city of Troy, perhaps during the Trojan War. Here are the rules:

• Each group of three chips of the same color can be replaced by a single token of this color in the square to the left.

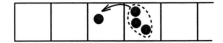

• Two different-colored tokens in the same square can be removed.

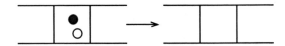

❖ From this starting position, find the minimum number of tokens and their positions at the end of the game.

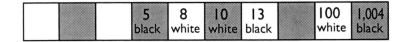

45 ❖ From Romeo to Juliet

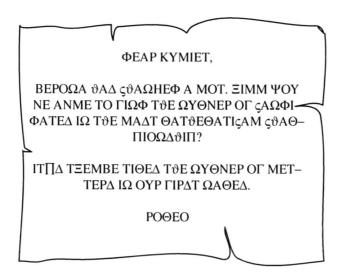

ΦΕΑΡ ΚΥΜΙΕΤ,

ΒΕΡΟΩΑ ϑΑΔ ςϑΑΩΗΕΦ Α ΜΟΤ. ΞΙΜΜ ΨΟΥ
ΝΕ ΑΝΜΕ ΤΟ ΓΙΩΦ ΤϑΕ ΩΥΘΝΕΡ ΟΓ ςΑΩΦΙ–
ΦΑΤΕΔ ΙΩ ΤϑΕ ΜΑΔΤ ΘΑΤϑΕΘΑΤΙςΑΜ ςϑΑΘ–
ΠΙΟΩΔϑΙΠ?

ΙΤΠΔ ΤΞΕΜΒΕ ΤΙΘΕΔ ΤϑΕ ΩΥΘΝΕΡ ΟΓ ΜΕΤ–
ΤΕΡΔ ΙΩ ΟΥΡ ΓΙΡΔΤ ΩΑΘΕΔ.

ΡΟΘΕΟ

❖ Give Juliet's answer to Romeo.

46 ❖ Nicholas's Watch

Nicholas has a digital watch. Each digit is shown with a certain number of liquid crystals (see Figure 1).

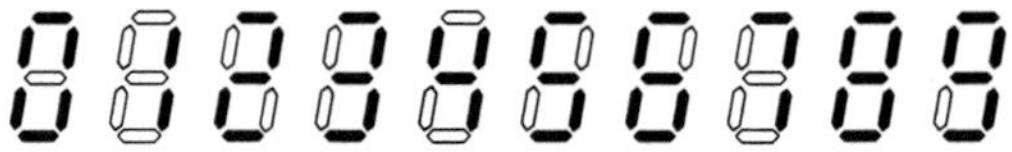

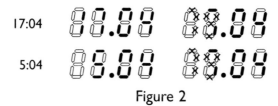

Figure 1

Twenty-four-hour time is displayed from 0:00 to 23:59. For the hours, the tens digit is shown only if it is not zero, while for the minutes, the tens digit is always shown. The left side of Figure 2 shows the watch times at 17:04 and 5:04.

17:04

5:04

Figure 2

Yet it is possible, as shown on the right side of Figure 2, that when some liquid crystals are not functional, Nicholas cannot distinguish 17:04 from 5:04.

❖ What is the maximum number of liquid crystals (horizontal and vertical) that can be nonfunctional so that Nicholas never has two different times displayed in the same way?

47 ❖ X Cannot Live There

The pentomino *X* cannot live in House 1, but it can live in House 2, as shown below. The pentomino's five squares coincide with squares of the house, and none of its squares is black.

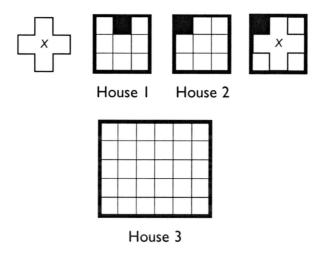

House 1   House 2

House 3

❖ What is the smallest number of black squares that we have to put inside House 3 so that *X* cannot live there?

48 ❖ A Little Logic

W alter claims:

    1. Of the three propositions A, B, and C, exactly one is true.
    2. Of the three propositions B, C, and D, exactly one is true.
    3. Of the two propositions A and D, exactly one is true.

Lydia claims:

    1. Of the three propositions A, B, and C, exactly one is true.
    2. Of the three propositions B, C, and D, exactly one is true.
    3. Of the three propositions A, C, and D, exactly one is true.

One of them is telling the truth and the other lies at least once.

❖ Put a check mark on each true proposition below.

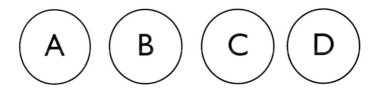

49 ❖ Master Fibo Unchains Himself

Master Fibo submitted the following request to his friend, a blacksmith:

"Here are ten chains. Two of them consist of a single link while the others are made up of 2, 3, 5, 8, 13, 21, 34, and 55 links. I would like you to assemble several chains, all having the same length, without making any loop."

It takes the blacksmith 1 minute to open and close a link.

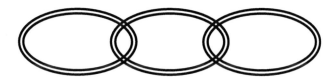

❖ What is the minimum time necessary to complete the job?

50 ❖ The Diamond

All the numbers between 1 and 14 are arranged in the circles of this beautiful diamond so that the difference between two numbers joined by a line always equals 1, 2, 4, or 5.

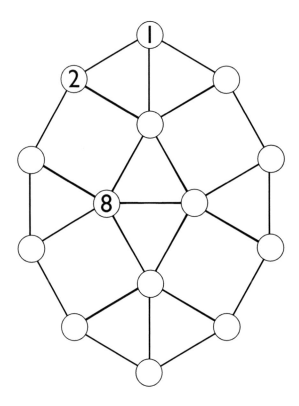

❖ Fill in the remaining circles.

1. The Eight Pieces

Here are **two solutions** for cutting up the hexagon into eight pieces, all the same size and shape:

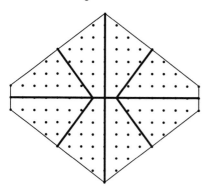

2. The Four Strings

First, consider two pieces of string tied together. If we pull these pieces to form two sides of a triangle, the greatest possible area is obtained when they are perpendicular; if $h < b$, we have $ah/2 < ab/2$. It is now easy to see that the four pieces of string have to be placed in two directions that are perpendicular to each other.

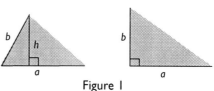

Figure I

There are three different ways to fulfill this requirement: The piece opposite the piece of length 3 can be of length 5 (Figure 2), of length 11 (Figure 3), or of length 13 (Figure 4).

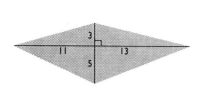

Figure 2

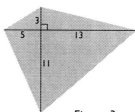

Figure 3

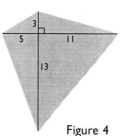

Figure 4

The area of Figure 2 is $(3 + 5)(11 + 13)/2 = 8 \times 24/2 = 96$ m^2.

The area of Figure 3 is $(3 + 11)(5 + 13)/2 = 14 \times 18/2 = 126$ m^2.

The area of Figure 4 is $(3 + 13)(5 + 11)/2 = 16 \times 16/2 = 128$ m^2.

The maximum possible area obtained by pulling the four strings tautly is **128 m^2.**

3. The Cut Square

Let *ABCD* be the square. Assume that the side cut into two segments of lengths 1 cm and 13 cm is $\overline{AB}$.

The perimeter has to be cut into two parts 35 cm and 21 cm long. Following the square clockwise, we can first find the 35-cm part (see Figure 1) or the 21-cm part (see Figure 2). We then verify that in both cases another side of the square has been cut into two parts 6 cm and 8 cm long; it is side $\overline{DC}$ in Figure 1 and side $\overline{BC}$ in Figure 2.

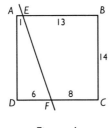

Figure 1

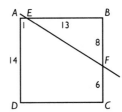

Figure 2

In the first case, the smaller area is equal to $14 \times (1 + 6)/2 = 49$ cm^2 (the area of trapezium *AEFD*).

In the second case, the smaller area is equal to $13 \times 8/2 = 52$ cm^2 (the area of triangle *EBF*).

This problem has two solutions: The area of the smaller part of the square equals either **49 cm^2** or **52 cm^2.**

4. Rose's Scarf

Triangle *ADI* has a right angle at *D*. So the angles at *A* and *I* are complementary and their tangents are inverse to each other. But tan $A = RE/AE = RE/12$ and tan $I = OS/SI = OS/27$. So $RE/12 = 27/OS$. It follows that $RE \times OS = 12 \times 27 = 324$. The product $RE \times OS$ is the area of the square *ROSE,* in cm^2. So, Rose's scarf cost **324 French Francs.**

5. Crosses on a Checkerboard

There are two different strategies. We can first try to cover the center of the checkerboard with the smallest possible number of cards and then cover the rest of the board. Alternatively, we can try to cover the border squares and finish the game in the center.

Surprisingly, the second strategy is the better one. We can cover the checkerboard using **9 cards.** There are only three such configurations with 9 cards: the symmetrical solution of Figure 1, and, because of symmetry about the center axis, the solution of Figure 2 and its reflection about the center axis.

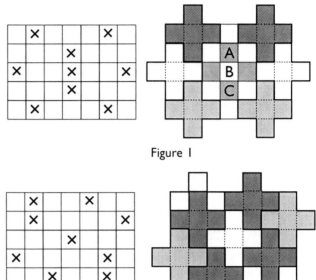

Figure I

Figure 2

6. Leo's Transmissions

It is convenient to identify the 12 pentominoes drawn here with the letters T, U, V, W, X, Y, Z, F, I, L, P, N:

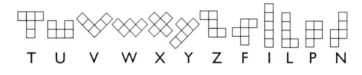

T   U   V   W   X   Y   Z   F   I   L   P   N

V, T, and P have already been used, so it remains to cover the grid with the 9 pentominoes U, W, X, Y, Z, F, I, L, and N. It is convenient to break up the grid into regions with a multiple of five squares, namely, regions *A, B,* and *C,* represented here:

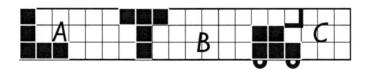

Region *C* must contain 10 squares. That precisely defines its frontier with region *B.* Looking over all the possibilities, it's clear that region *C* can be filled only with pentominoes U and X.

To avoid too many attempts, let's now try to place the W. It can go into region *A* or region *B* adjacent to the T, and these are the only possibilities; in the other cases, the W cuts one of these regions into areas that are not multiples of 5. If we put the W in region *A*, as just suggested, then it's impossible to complete the filling up. If we put the W in region *B*, then the problem has a solution: Put the F in *A*, then the L and the N in *A*, and, finally, put the I, Y, and Z in *B*.

From this we get **the unique solution** shown below.

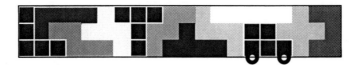

7. Four Colors for a Coloring

First, notice that 3 black centers (Bk in the figure) are already in the square. So the last black center is in c3. Since this square cannot have a black border, the squares d3 and c1 must have a black border. On the bottom row, the red center must be in c1, and on the previous row it is in b2. Then a red center has to be placed on the last column; it must be in d3. So there is a white center in a1. A red border has to be either in a1 and b3, or in a3 and b1, but, since we cannot have white-white on a1, the red border must be in a1 and b3.

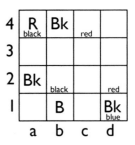

	a	b	c	d
4	R black	Bk	red	
3				
2	Bk	black		red
1		B		Bk blue

The rest of the figure follows easily: blue center in a3, white border in a3, blue border in c3, white border in c2, blue border in a2, white border in d4, blue border in b4, white border in b1, white center in d2, blue center in c2, white center in c4, white center in b3, and blue center in d4.

We obtain **the unique solution** shown here.

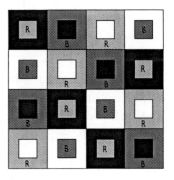

8. The Three-Colored Knights

Let 1, 2, 3 be the three colors, and let *a, b, c, d, e, f* be the six regions to color. First, notice that region *a* has to be colored with color 1 or 3 (since it is connected with a region whose color is 2). In the same way, region *d* has to be colored with

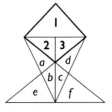

color 1 or 2. Looking at the sequence a, b, c, d, we have to build all the sequences of the following types:

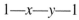

1—x—y—1
1—x—y—2
3—x—y—1
3—x—y—2

where x is different from the first number, x is different from y, and y is different from the last number. There are 11 such sequences:

1—2—1—2
1—2—3—1
1—2—3—2
1—3—1—2
1—3—2—1
3—1—2—1
3—1—3—1
3—1—3—2
3—2—1—2
3—2—3—1
3—2—3—2

We check that there is only one way of coloring the regions e and f. So the knight's country has **11 counties,** as shown here.

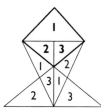
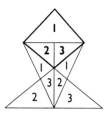
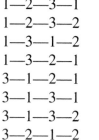
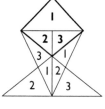
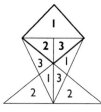
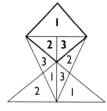
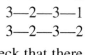
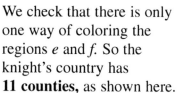
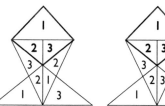
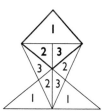

9. The Four-Color Process

In this figure, we represent the colors as given by the data, layer by layer. It is easy to fill in the third layer. Square 1 has **W** and **B** to its left and right and **V** in front of it, so it can only be **G**.

Square 2 must be **V**. In the same way, Square 3, being aligned with **W**, **G**, and **V**, must contain **B**; that fills squa-

V	W	B	G
G	B	W	V
B	G	V	W
W	V	G	B

Layer 4

W	2	1	B
8	6	3	W
7	5	4	V
B	W	V	G

Layer 3

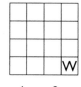

Layer 2

Layer 1

re 4 with a **B**. **W** must
be in square 5 and **G** in square 6. Square 7 is **G**
and square 8 is **V**.

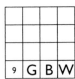 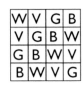 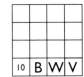

In Layers 1 and 2, we have
to work on vertical columns,
using the already filled last
two layers. We then find
that 9 is **V** and 10 is **G**.

So all the squares are logical-
ly filled one after
the other and we obtain
the solution shown here.

V	W	B	G
G	B	W	V
B	G	V	W
W	V	G	B

Layer 4

W	V	G	B
V	G	B	W
G	B	W	V
B	W	V	G

Layer 3

G	B	W	V
B	W	V	G
W	V	G	B
V	G	B	W

Layer 2

B	G	V	W
W	V	G	B
V	W	B	G
G	B	W	V

Layer 1

10. Surrounding 55

First we note that $1,980 = 36 \times 55$. Then we look at all the
possible factorizations of 36 with two factors:

$36 = 1 \times 36$ $36 = 2 \times 18$ $36 = 3 \times 12$
$36 = 4 \times 9$ $36 = 6 \times 6$

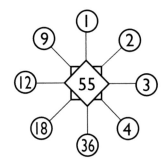

This last product cannot work, since the eight numbers have
to be different. So there are four possible decompositions,
since we have four different three-number rows.

We have $1 + 2 + 3 + 4 + 9 + 12 + 18 + 36 = 85$.
The sum of the eight numbers surrounding 55 is then **85.**

11. Matthew and Multiples

The sum of the twelve numbers in Grandpa Joss's
array is $108 + 35 + 42 + 97 + 120 + 70 +$
$216 + 175 + 294 + 197 + 240 + 70 = 1,664$.

So, Grandpa will give Matthew 1,664 French Francs
for finding all the numbers.

Then Matthew will give Matilda half of the award, so
she will earn 1,664/2, that is, **832 French Francs.**

The nearest number to 95							The nearest number to 196
a	2	3	4	5	7	9	b
108	yes	yes	yes	no	no	yes	216
35	no	no	no	yes	yes	no	175
42	yes	yes	no	no	yes	no	294
97	no	no	no	no	no	no	197
120	yes	yes	yes	yes	no	no	240
70	yes	no	no	yes	yes	no	70

Divisible by

12. Truncadivisible

One-digit numbers cannot be truncadivisible since, if we remove the last digit, then nothing remains.

Let us look at two-digit numbers.

All the numbers beginning with 1 are truncadivisible. There are 10 numbers from 10 to 19. All the even numbers beginning with 2 are truncadivisible: 20, 22, 24, 26, 28 (5 numbers). Among all the numbers with a tens digit greater than 2, we get 30, 33, 36, 39 (4 numbers), 40, 44, 48 (3 numbers), 50, 55, 60, 66, 70, 77, 80, 88, 90, and 99 (10 numbers).

Let's look at the numbers greater than 99.

Let n be such a number. We write $n = 10t + u$, where $u < 10$.

In this formula, u is the units digit of n and t is a number with at least two digits, representing how many multiples of ten n contains.

So n is truncadivisible if and only if t divides into n. Since t divides into $10t$, we conclude that t divides into u. Since t is (strictly) greater than u, then u must be 0. So the numbers greater than 99 that are truncadivisible exactly are the multiples of 10. From 100 to 1,995, there are 190 multiples of 10 (from 10×10 to 199×10). So the total number of truncadivisible numbers from 10 to 1,995 is

$10 + 5 + 4 + 3 + 10 + 190 = $ **222 truncadivisible numbers.**

13. The Karr Brothers

First method:

We need to find n consecutive integers whose sum is 1,995. Let a be the smallest integer. We have

$$a + (a + 1) + (a + 2) + \cdots + (a + n - 1) = 1,995$$
$$na + n(n - 1)/2 = 1,995$$

From this, we have $a = 1,995/n - (n - 1)/2$.

Since a is an integer, we have two possibilities:

1. n is an odd number that divides 1,995 exactly, so $(n - 1)/2$ is an integer and so is a.
2. n is an even number, so $1,995/n$ and $(n - 1)/2$ are not integers, but $a = 1,995/n - (n - 1)/2$ is an integer because the decimal parts of the quotients cancel each other out.

Let's express 1,995 as the product of its prime factors: $1,995 = 3 \times 5 \times 7 \times 19$.

So n has four possibilities: 3, 5, 7, and 6 (3×2), all the other possibilities being greater than 9 or equal to 2.

$n = 3$ gives the answer $a = 665 - 1 = 664$,
$n = 5$ gives the answer $a = 399 - 2 = 397$,
$n = 7$ gives the answer $a = 285 - 3 = 282$, and
$n = 6$ gives the answer $a = 332.5 - 2.5 = 330$.

So this problem has **4 solutions:** the least wealthy Karr brother has **282 sheep, 330 sheep, 397 sheep,** or **664 sheep.**

Second method:
The sum of the integers from 1 to n is equal to $n(n + 1)/2 = (n^2 + n)/2$. So the sum of the integers from $m + 1$ to n is $(n^2 + n - m^2 - m)/2 = (n - m)(n + m + 1)/2$. So we have the equation $(n - m)(n + m + 1) = 2 \times 1{,}995 = 3{,}990$. But $3{,}990 = 1 \times 3{,}990 = 2 \times 1{,}995 = 3 \times 1{,}330 = 5 \times 798 = 6 \times 665 = 7 \times 570 = 10 \times 399 = 14 \times 285 = 19 \times 210 = 21 \times 150$. For all these factorizations, $3{,}990 = a \times b$, we solve the equations $n - m = a, n + m + 1 = b$. The conditions $n - m > 2, n - m < 10$, n and m integers, lead to four solutions: $m = 663$, $n = 666$; $m = 396, n = 401$; $m = 329, n = 335$; and $m = 281, n = 288$. The values of $m + 1$ give the same answers as found by the first method.

14. Little House on the Prairie

In one hour, Dad and Grandpa are able to dig $1/6 + 1/10 = 16/60$ of the garden. So the whole garden will be dug in

$$\frac{1}{\frac{16}{60}} = \frac{60}{16} = \frac{15}{4} = 3\frac{3}{4} \text{ hours, or } \mathbf{225 \text{ minutes}}$$

15. Of Dice and Decimals

We can forget about denominators of 3 and 6 as they give only three decimal numbers—1, 2, and 1/2—which can also be obtained with a denominator of 2.

- Denominator 5: The six numerators give decimal results.
- Denominator 4: All six numerators also give decimal results, but we can forget about 4/4, since 1 was previously obtained. So it gives five new results.
- Denominator 2: Three new decimal results with the numerators 4, 5, and 6.
- Denominator 1: Three new decimal results with the numerators 4, 5, and 6.

The total number of different terminating decimal results is then **17.**

16. Stacking Fractions

If we transform the stack into a simple fraction—for instance, with a single fraction line—the numerator and the denominator are products of numbers from the set {1, 2, 3, 4, 5, 6, 7, 8}, each of these numbers appearing once in either the numerator or the denominator. Moreover, 1 must be in the numerator and 2 in the denominator. Let's show that the other factors can be in the numerator or denominator independently of one another, depending on the order of divisions indicated by the size of the fraction lines.

Let n be an integer such that $3 \leq n \leq 8$. Consider the initial part of the stack that consists of the numbers from 1 to n with their corresponding fraction lines. Then n is guaranteed to be in the numerator of the simplified fraction if the line just above n is the largest in the complex fraction, and n is guaranteed to be in the denominator if the line just above $n - 1$ is the largest and the line just above n is the smallest.

Thus, each of the numbers from 3 to 8 can be in either the numerator or the denominator. This gives $2^6 = 64$ possibilities.

We now have to eliminate the possibilities that give the same results.

The equality $3 \times 8 = 4 \times 6$ implies that fractions of the forms

$$\frac{1 \times \cdots \times 3 \times 8}{2 \times \cdots \times 4 \times 6} \text{ and } \frac{1 \times \cdots \times 4 \times 6}{2 \times \cdots \times 3 \times 8}$$

give the same result. Since the positions of 1 and 2 are fixed, this equality is the only possible one. There are four such fractions since each of the remaining numbers, 5 and 7, can be in either the numerator or the denominator.

So we obtain $64 - 4 = $ **60 different results.**

17. Palindrome

The palindromes following 83338 are 83438, 83538, 83638, 83738, 83838, 83938, 84048, 84148, 84248, ...

The seventh palindrome after 83338 is **84048.**

18. The Quasi-Perfect Years

By deleting the first digit (1), we are in the 900s, among which are two perfect squares, 900 and 961. They lead to the solutions 1900 and 1961.

By deleting the second digit (9), we get a three-digit number beginning with 1. We get 1900, 1921, 1944, 1969, and 1996 (already found, and not smaller than 1996 anyway).

By deleting the third digit, we obtain "19a6," where a is any value from 0 to 8: 1906, 1916, 1926, 1936, 1946, 1956, 1966, 1976, 1986.

In the same way, deleting the fourth digit, we obtain "196b," where b is any value from 0 to 9: 1960, 1961, 1962, 1963, 1964, 1965, 1966, 1967, 1968, 1969.

Before 1996, in the 1900s, there were **21 quasi-perfect years:** 1900, 1906, 1916, 1921, 1926, 1936, 1944, 1946, 1956, 1960, 1961, 1962, 1963, 1964, 1965, 1966, 1967, 1968, 1969, 1976, and 1986.

19. Heads or Tails?

In the figure, the upper side of each of the four coins at each step is shown, indicating the coins that will be turned over on the next move.

We see that at the end of the eighth move the coins are in the starting position; the ninth move will be like the first one. So the moves form a cycle with period 8.

Since $1{,}995 = 8 \times 249 + 3$, after the 1,995th move the position will be the same as after the third move, namely, **tails, heads, tails, heads.**

Starting position	(H) (H) (H) (H)		
1st move	(T) (H) (H) (H)		
2nd move	(H) (T) (H) (H)		
3rd move	(T) (H) (T) (H)		
4th move	(H) (T) (H) (T)		
5th move	(T) (T) (H) (T)		
6th move	(H) (H) (H) (T)		
7th move	(T) (T) (T) (T)		
8th move	(H) (H) (H) (H)		

20. Sommersby

We begin by computing the first few rounds.

After the 15th round, there are no more blue soldiers (one was eliminated on each of the previous rounds).

After that 15th round, 80 orange soldiers and 126 green soldiers remain, including the multiple reinforcements. As the exercise continues, two green soldiers will be eliminated for every orange soldier, because there are no blue soldiers left. Since $126/2 = 63$ is smaller than 80, we conclude that eliminating the green and blue team will take $63 + 15 =$ **78 rounds** and that $80 - 63 =$ **17 soldiers of the orange team** will be left.

	Orange	Green	Blue
Starting position	95	51	15
1st round	94		14
2nd round	93		13
3rd round	92		12
4th round	91		11
5th round	90		10
6th round	89		9
7th round	88		8
8th round	87		7
9th round	86		6
10th round	85		5
11th round	84		4
12th round	83		3
13th round	82		2
14th round	81		1
15th round	80	126	0
16th round	79	124	0

21. The Magic Wheel

Call the seven numbers a, b, c, d, e, f, and g, as shown below.

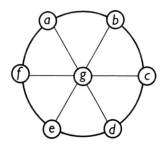

The sums of all three rows being equal, we can say that $a + d = b + e = c + f$. So we have $a + b + c + d + e + f + g = 3(a + d) + g$.

The sum of the numbers up to 7 is equal to $(7 \times 8)/2 = 28$. Putting together these two results, we deduce that $28 - g$ has to be a multiple of 3.

We can have $28 - 1 = 3 \times 9$, $28 - 4 = 3 \times 8$, and $28 - 7 = 3 \times 7$.

These equations lead to the three possibilities shown at right. So there are three solutions: The number in the center square is **1, 4,** or **7.**

① 2 3 4 5 6 7

1 2 3 ④ 5 6 7

1 2 3 4 5 6 ⑦

22. Missing Numbers

From the data and the partly filled-in table, it is easy to see that $f = 2$ or 3, $e = 2$ or 3, $h = 7$ or 9, and $c = 7$ or 9.

×	c	d	5	e
f		12		6
g		24		A
8			40	
h	63	B		

Assuming that $f = 2$, then $e = 3$, $d = 6$, $g = 4$, and $A = 12$. Depending on whether $h = 7$ or 9, $B = 42$ or $B = 54$.

If we assume that $f = 3$, then $e = 2$, $d = 4$, $g = 6$, and $A = 12$ (as in the first case). Depending on whether $h = 7$ or 9, $B = 28$ or $B = 36$.

So the possible values of B are **28, 36, 42,** and **54.** The four corresponding tables are shown below.

×	9	4	5	2
3	27	12	15	6
6	54	24	30	12
8	72	32	40	16
7	63	**28**	35	14

×	9	6	5	3
2	18	12	10	6
4	36	24	20	12
8	72	48	40	24
7	63	**42**	35	21

×	7	4	5	2
3	21	12	15	6
6	42	24	30	12
8	56	32	40	16
9	63	**36**	45	18

×	7	6	5	3
2	14	12	10	6
4	28	24	20	12
8	56	48	40	24
9	63	**54**	45	27

23. The Raffle

Bob said 4; so his cards must be numbered 1 and 3.

David said $7 = 1 + 6 = 2 + 5 = 3 + 4$. Bob already has cards 1 and 3, so David has the cards numbered 2 and 5.

Alice said $11 = 10 + 1 = 9 + 2 = 8 + 3 = 7 + 4 = 6 + 5$. The cards 1, 2, 3, and 5 already belong to someone else, so Alice must have cards 4 and 7.

Chris said $16 = 12 + 4 = 11 + 5 = 10 + 6 = 9 + 7$. The cards 4, 5, and 7 already belong to someone else, so Chris must have cards 6 and 10.

The remaining cards are 8, 9, 11, and 12. To obtain 19 as a sum, we have to choose cards 8 and 11. So Elizabeth has these two.

The problem has only one solution:
Alice, 4; Bob, 1; Chris, 6; David, 2; and Elizabeth, 8.

24. The Nine Numbers

The number situated in the ith row and the jth column has the value

$9(i - 1) + j$, if i is odd

or $9(i - 1) + (10 - j)$, if i is even.

1	2	3	4	⑤	6	7	8	9
18	17	16	⑮	14	13	12	11	10
19	20	21	22	23	㉔	25	26	27
36	35	㉞	33	32	31	30	29	28
37	38	39	40	41	42	㊸	44	45
54	㊼	52	51	50	49	48	47	46
55	56	57	58	59	60	61	㊽	63
㊺	71	70	69	68	67	66	65	64
73	74	75	76	77	78	79	80	㊶

To obtain the maximum possible sum, we need to minimize the value of j in the even rows and maximize this value in the odd rows. We get this maximum by taking j in the set $\{1, 2, 3, 4\}$ for $i = 2, 4, 6$, and 8 and j in the set $\{5, 6, 7, 8, 9\}$ for $i = 1, 3, 5, 7$, and 9.

We then obtain the sum:

$0 + 5 + 9 + (10 - 1) + 18 + 6 + 27 + (10 - 2) + 36 + 7 + 45 + (10 - 3) + 54 + 8 + 63 + (10 - 4) + 72 + 9 = 5 + 18 + 24 + 35 + 43 + 52 + 62 + 69 + 81 = 389.$

The maximum possible value of the sum of the nine numbers is **389.**

Alternative method:

First, fill the whole array. Begin with the greatest number in the array and erase the numbers in its row and column. Repeat the previous step with the remaining 8×8 array, then with the remaining 7×7 array, and so on.

We then obtain $81 + 72 + 62 + 53 + 43 + 34 + 24 + 15 + 5 = $ **389.**

This method does not guarantee obtaining the maximum possible value, but it works quite well in practice.

25. Ninety-nine

Putting in 8 plus signs, that is, as many plus signs as possible, we obtain the sum

$$1 + 2 + 3 + 4 + 5 + 6 + 7 + 8 + 9 = 45$$

Let's see what happens if we remove only one plus sign. If we remove the first plus sign, we replace $1 + 2$ by 12, so the total sum increases by $12 - (1 + 2) = 9$. In the same way, if we remove the second plus sign, the total sum increases by $23 - (2 + 3) = 18$. In the figure on the next page, we can see how the total sum increases with the removal of the corresponding plus sign.

$$+\ 9 \uparrow \quad +18 \uparrow \quad +27 \uparrow \quad +36 \uparrow \quad +45 \uparrow \quad +54 \uparrow \quad +63 \uparrow \quad +72 \uparrow$$

It is obvious that if we removed two consecutive plus signs, we would obtain a three-digit number, making it impossible to reach 99.

Removing two (or more) nonconsecutive plus signs makes the sum increase by the amount of each increment.

The problem is now equivalent to reaching 99 from 45 by adding numbers taken in the sequence (9, 18, 27, 36, 45, 54, 63, 72) without taking two consecutive ones.

There are **three solutions:**

$$99 = 45 + 54$$
$$99 = 45 + 45 + 9$$
$$99 = 45 + 36 + 18$$

These three solutions correspond to the **three sums:**

$$\mathbf{1 + 2 + 3 + 4 + 5 + 67 + 8 + 9 = 99}$$
$$\mathbf{12 + 3 + 4 + 56 + 7 + 8 + 9 = 99}$$
$$\mathbf{1 + 23 + 45 + 6 + 7 + 8 + 9 = 99}$$

26. The Compact Disk

Let x be the price of the CD in French Francs.

First, we know that $x > 47$, since Matthew is 47 French Francs short and his piggy bank is not empty. Moreover, $(x - 47) + (x - 2) < x$, since, putting their money together, they cannot buy the CD. This inequality reduces to $x < 49$.

From these inequalities, $x > 47$ and $x < 49$, there is only one solution, $x = 48$.

So the price of the CD is **48 French Francs.**

27. Full House

Let g be the number of girls in this family (including Jenny), and let b be the number of boys (including Jim).

Jenny is the sixth child, so this family has at least six children, and $b + g \geq 6$. Jenny has at least as many brothers as sisters, leading to $b \geq g - 1$. Jim has at least twice as many sisters as brothers, giving $g \geq 2 (b - 1)$.

From $b \geq g - 1$, we conclude that $b - g \geq -1$. Adding this result to $b + g \geq 6$, we conclude that $2b \geq 5$, or $b \geq 5/2$.

From $g \geq 2b - 2$, we conclude that $-2b + g \geq -2$. Adding this result to $b - g \geq -1$, we conclude that $-b \geq -3$, or $b \leq 3$.

Since b must be a whole number, we conclude that $b = 3$.

Combining this result with $b \geq g - 1$ we conclude that $g \leq 4$, and combining it with $g \geq 2(b - 1)$ we conclude that $g \geq 4$.

Thus, we conclude that $g = 4$.

There are **4 girls and 3 boys** in Jenny and Jim's family.

28. Where's He From?

Let "ab" be the number, where a and b are its digits: $0 < a \leq 9$ and $0 < b \leq 9$.

We have the equation $94 - (10a + b) = a + b$, which leads to $11a + 2b = 94$. From this last equation, we see that a is even. We can study all the possibilities, according to the value of a (0, 2, 4, 6, or 8):

a	0	2	4	6	8
$11a$	0	22	44	66	88
b	47	36	25	14	3

Only when a is 8 will b be smaller than 10 (b is the units digit of the number, so it is less than 10).

So the number is **83.**

29. Encyclonumberist

Since the left page number is even, the tens and hundreds digits of both pages must be the same.

These two numbers are of the form "abc" and "ab(c + 1)." The sum of the digits of these two numbers equals 25, so we have $2(a + b + c) + 1 = 25$, which simplifies to $a + b + c = 12$.

Since a, b, and c are consecutive, they belong to the set $\{3, 4, 5\}$. The only even digit is 4, so we conclude that $c = 4$. The units digit of the left page is 4 and that of the right page is 5.

So there are two solutions, namely, **354** and **534.**

30. Maggie's Birth Month

Translating the steps of the problem, we get $4x + (12 - x) - 2(5 + x) = 10$.
Simplifying gives $x + 2 = 10$ or $x = 8$.
So Maggie's birth month is **August.**

31. An Interesting Property

Mr. Gideon's property is a 28-sided polygon. Since the sides have the same length, let L be that length so that the perimeter of the property is $28L$.

Because the polygon contains 25 squares, it is easy to see that the area of the property is equal to $25L^2$.

Since the perimeter is equal to the area, we have $25L^2 = 28L$, from which we get $L(25L - 28) = 0$ and then $25L = 28$ (since $L > 0$).

So $L = 28/25 = 1.12$ km $= 1,120$ m.

So the perimeter of the property is equal to $1,120 \times 28 = $ **31,360 meters.**

32. Numerical Polygons

Let's study each circuit independently.

On the square-shaped circuit, let x be the content of the left upper corner.

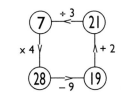

Following the circuit, we conclude that $(4x - 7)/3 = x$, which has the unique solution $x = 7$. So we can complete the whole circuit.

On the second circuit, let x be the content of the left upper corner. This leads to the equation $2((x - 17)/7 + 16) = x$, which has the unique solution $x = 38$. So we can complete the whole circuit.

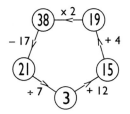

On the third circuit, let x be the content of the left upper corner. This leads to the equation $3((x/2 + 44)/3 - 5) - 10 = x$, which has the unique solution $x = 38$. So we can complete the whole circuit.

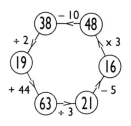

Two numbers appear three times: 19 and 21. So the problem has two solutions. Therefore, Kevin and Diana Jones must press **the stones numbered 19** or **the stones numbered 21.**

---

50 Mathematical Puzzles and Problems ◆ *Orange Collection*
©2001 Key Curriculum Press

33. The Lucky Year

First method:

The thousands digit of the lucky year is 1. Let a be its hundreds digit, and let X be the two-digit number formed with its last two digits.

The following equation holds and reduces as follows:

$$2X(10 + a) = 1{,}000 + 100a + X$$
$$19X + 2a(X - 50) = 1{,}000$$
$$19(X - 50) + 2a(X - 50) = 50$$
$$(19 + 2a)(X - 50) = 50$$

The only possible odd value for $19 + 2a$ is 25, which gives $a = 3$ and $X = 52$.

The lucky year was **1352.**

Second method:

Let "1xyz," that is, $1{,}000 + 100x + 10y + z$, be the lucky year. We have "yz" $\times$ "1x" $\times 2 =$ "1xyz," that is, $(10y + z)(10 + x) + 2 = 1{,}000 + 100x + 10y + z$. So z must be even, and we have $200y + 20xy + 20z + 2xz = 1{,}000 + 100x + 10y + z$, which rearranges to $2xz - z = 1{,}000 + 100x - 190y - 20xy - 20z$, which factors to $z(2x - 1) = 10(100 + 10x - 19y - 2xy - 2z)$, so $z(2x - 1)$ is divisible by 10. Since z cannot be at the same time even and a multiple of 5, we deduce that $2x - 1$ is divisible by 5.

The case $x = 3$ leads to the solution **1352,** while the case $x = 8$ leads to nowhere.

Third method:

Let X be the two-digit number formed with the first two digits of the lucky year, and let Y be the number formed with its last two digits. We have $100X + Y = 2XY$, where X and Y are greater than 0.

So we deduce that $100 + (Y/X) = 2Y$. Thus, Y/X is an integer.

So we must have $Y = kX$, where k is a positive integer.

From the first equation divided by Y, we deduce that $100/k + 1 = 2X$.

So k has to be a divisor of 100; also, $100/k$ must be odd.

$k = 20$ gives $X = 3$ and $Y = 60$, which does not work (0360).

$k = 4$ gives $X = 13$ and $Y = 52$, leading to the solution **1352.**

Fourth method:

Let X be the two-digit number formed with the first two digits of the lucky year, and let Y be the number formed with its last two digits. We have $100X + Y = 2XY$, so $2X(Y - 50) = Y$. Thus, Y is greater than 50 and $2X$ is greater than or equal to 20. The only case that satisfies both conditions is $Y = 52$, which gives $X = 13$, and the solution **1352**.

34. Diana Jones's Suitcase

Let c be the number of crabs and s the number of spiders. We have $10c + 8s = 28$, which simplifies to $5c + 4s = 14$. $0 \le 5c \le 14$, so $0 \le c \le 2$, since c must be an integer.

c cannot be 0 since 14 is not a multiple of 4; nor can c equal 1, for a similar reason. If $c = 2$, then $s = 1$, the remaining 4 heads being the heads of the snakes.

Diana Jones has in her suitcase **4 snakes, 1 spider, and 2 crabs.**

35. The Great Current

Let b be the speed of the barge, and let c be the speed of the current.

We have

$$2(b + c) = 60 \qquad \text{(going down the river)}$$
$$3(b - c) = 60 \qquad \text{(going up the river)}$$

Solving these equations gives $b = 25$ and $c = 5$. The speed of the current is **5 km/h.**

36. The Three Couples

Let a, b, c, d, e, and f be the respective ages of Alice, Betty, Carolyn, Dan, Earl, and Frank. We know that $a + b + c + d + e + f = 137$.

All men being five years older than their wives, the equation reduces to $(2a + 5) + (2b + 5) + (2c + 5) = 137$. Betty and her husband are 47 years old together, so we deduce that $b = 21$ and $e = 26$. The previous equation now reduces to $2a + 2c = 80$, or $a + c = 40$.

If Betty is the youngest woman, then either a or $c = 21 + 4 = 25$. In either case, the other is 15, contradicting the hypothesis. So the oldest is Alice and the youngest is Carolyn.

So $a = c + 4$, and we deduce that $a = 22$ and $c = 18$. It is then easy to compute the age of each man.

Dan is 27, Earl is 26, and Frank is 23.

---

37. The V.H.L.

At the beginning, Milo is at the 0th rung. Just before his second jump, he will be at the $(13 - 1)$th rung. Just before his third jump, he will be at the $(13 - 1) + (13 - 2)$th rung. More generally, just before his $(n + 1)$st jump, he will be at rung number $(13 - 1) + (13 - 2) + (13 - 3) + \cdots + (13 - n)$.

To reach the floor after n jumps, this number has to be smaller than or equal to zero: $(13 - 1) + (13 - 2) + (13 - 3) + \cdots + (13 - n) \leq 0$.

The equation reduces to $13n - n(n + 1)/2 \leq 0$, leading to $n(25 - n) \leq 0$.

The only solutions are 25 or more (for $n > 0$).

So Milo will reach the floor after **25 jumps.**

38. Lucy's Laces

The following table summarizes all the results.

	After school	Once at home
Monday	2 double knots, 0 single knots	2 double knots
Tuesday	3 double knots, 1 single knot	3 double knots
Thursday	4 double knots, 1 single knot	4 double knots
Friday	2 double knots, 1 single knot	2 double knots

On Friday night, at home, two double knots remained, that is, **four knots** on Lucy's laces.

39. Sum Up the Neighbors

When the number 1 is put in a, the number 2 can be in c, d, or e. Since e is then symmetrical to c about the a-d axis, we can forget about the case $e = 2$ and consider only the case $c = 2$, temporarily ignoring the condition $b < f$. If we then get a configuration where $b > f$, we simply take the mirror image of the configuration, reflected across the a-d axis.

Let's try to place the integers 2 to 6 with the condition that two consecutive numbers are not in adjacent positions.

The case where 2 is in d: Then 3 can be in *b* or *f.* Since *b* < *f,* 3 has to be in *b*. The number 5 must be in *c*, and 4 and 6 are in the two remaining positions. So there are two distinct possibilities (A and B).

 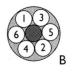

The case where 2 is in c: Then 3 can be in *e* or *f.* First, let's assume that 3 is in *e*. Then 4 is in *b*, and 5 and 6 are in the two remaining positions. So there are two distinct possibilities (C and D). If 3 is in *f,* then 4 cannot be in *b,* since that would force 5 and 6 to be adjacent. Therefore 4 must be in *d,* and either 5 is in *b* and 6 is in *e* or vice versa (E and F). However, these give *b* > *f,* so we take their mirror images across the *a-d* axis (G and H). We now have to check that it is possible to compute all the scores from 1 to 21 using A, B, C, D, G, and H. Since the balls are in a circle, if we obtain a score, we can also obtain the difference between this score and 21: We take the remaining balls, which must be adjacent. So we only have to check the scores from 0 to 10. 0 is easy: We don't take any balls. The numbers from 1 to 6 are also easily obtained by taking the corresponding single ball. We then check that all the scores from 7 to 10 can be obtained with each of the six configura-

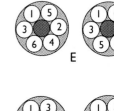

tions. So all the scores can be obtained with all the configurations; there are **six solutions:**

40. Doubly True

Smallest value of ONZE:

To get the smallest value of ONZE, we first choose the smallest possible values for C and O, namely, C = 1 and O = 2. We know that S + I ≥ 9 since there is a carry. Once again, we choose the smallest possible value, N = 0. From this, we get Z = I + 1 and S + I = 10. There are four possibilities for (S, I, Z), namely, (7, 3, 4), (6, 4, 5), (4, 6, 7), and (3, 7, 8). The first triplet minimizes the value of ONZE.

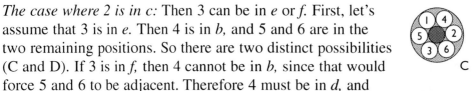

$$\begin{array}{r} S\ I\ X \\ +\ 1\ I\ N\ Q \\ \hline 2\ N\ Z\ E \end{array}$$

The remaining digits for X, Q, and E are 5, 6, 8, and 9. Since X + Q = 10 + E, the only possibility is 9 + 6 = 10 + 5 (the roles of X and Q being interchangeable).

```
    7 3 9
+   1 3 0 6
  ─────────
    2 0 4 5
```

The **smallest value** of ONZE is **2,045.**

Greatest value of ONZE:

In this case, we choose the largest possible values for C and O, namely, C = 8 and O = 9.

```
      S I X
+   8 I N Q
  ─────────
    9 N Z E
```

The greatest possible value for S + I is 7 + 6 = 13, possibly incremented if the previous sum is greater than 10. If we assume that this occurs, we get N = 4. It is clearly better to have I = 7 and S = 6 since that maximizes Z.

The remaining digits are 5, 3, 2, 1, and 0.
So X + Q < 10 and Z = 1.

The only possibility for the units digits is 3 + 2 = 5, or 2 + 3 = 5.

```
      6 7 X
+   8 7 4 Q
  ─────────
    9 4 1 5
```

The **greatest value** of ONZE is **9,415.**

41. Taking Photos

Each person must appear on at least two photos: one for each of the friends that appears with him on the first photo (since those two friends cannot choose photos of themselves). Thus, the number of photos must be greater than or equal to $2n$, where n is the number of people.

Let p be the number of photos. There are $3p$ photographed people. As seen previously, we must have $3p \geq 2n$. In our case, we obtain $3p \geq 18$, so $p \geq 6$.

There *is* a solution with 6 photos: Place the nine friends in a 3×3 square and take for the photos the rows and columns of this square. Each friend will have to choose the four photos in which he doesn't appear.

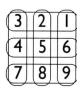

Consistent with the requirements, the minimum number of photos of the nine friends is therefore **6.**

Note: There are many different solutions, but it can be proved that they all are equivalent, merely being renumberings of the nine friends.

42. Drawing Straws

Let *a, b, c, d,* and *e* be the bets of Allen, Bob, Chris, Dan, and Edward, respectively, where $a > b > c > d > e$.

Let us define *Z* as the player who lost the last game, *Y* as the player who lost the next-to-last game, *X* as the player who lost the third game, *W* as the player who lost the second game, and *V* as the player who lost the first game.

Let's do a backward analysis, that is, examine the credits of each player from the end of the last game back to the beginning bets.

We then deduce that $A = V$, $B = W$, $C = X$, $D = Y$, and $E = Z$. So the initial bets of each player were, respectively, **81, 41, 21, 11, and 6 French Francs.**

	V	W	X	Y	Z
After the fifth game	32	32	32	32	32
After the fourth game	16	16	16	16	96
After the third game	8	8	8	88	48
After the second game	4	4	84	44	24
After the first game	2	82	42	22	12
Initial bets	81	41	21	11	6

43. The Willows

On the last move, 5 sparrows move from the fifth willow to the first. So there are at least 5 sparrows in the first willow at the end, meaning at least 5 sparrows in *every* willow, meaning at least 25 sparrows in all.

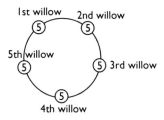

Since there cannot be 6 in each tree (the total number of sparrows is smaller than 30), there are exactly 25 sparrows.

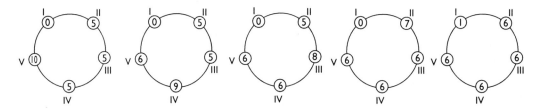

Doing a backward analysis, that is, working from the last move to the first, we find that the five willows had, before their dance, **1 sparrow, 6 sparrows, 6 sparrows, 6 sparrows, and 6 sparrows.**

44. Troy Moves

Clearly the rules can be applied in any order without changing the final result.

We'll play the game from the rightmost square to the leftmost square and always apply the second rule before the first one.

The minimum number of tokens remaining is **4,** with the positions as shown.

		5 black	8 white	10 white	13 black	100 white	1,004 black
		5 black	8 white	10 white	13 black	100 w 334 b	2 b
		5 black	8 white	10 white	13 black	234 b	2 b
		5 black	8 white	10 white	13 black	78 b	2 b
		5 black	8 white	10 white	13b 26b		2 b
		5 black	8 white	10w 13b			2 b
		5 black	8 white	3 b			2 b
		5 black	8w 1b				2 b
		5 black	7w				2 b
		5b 2w	1w				2 b
		3b	1w				2 b
		b	w				2 b

45. From Romeo to Juliet

It is easy to find the beginning "Dear Juliet," the signature "Romeo," and the word "mathematical." Then we obtain the coding of the 11 letters: A, C, D, E, H, I, L, M, R, T, and U. The remaining part of the message decodes easily:

Dear Juliet,

Verona has changed a lot.

Will you be able to find the number of candidates in the last mathematical championship?

It's twelve times the number of letters in our first names.

Romeo

"Romeo" has 5 letters and "Juliet" has 6, so the sum is 11.
Twelve times this sum is 132.

Juliet's answer to Romeo is **132.**

46. Nicholas's Watch

To be able to tell the time without ambiguity, there must be no doubt about each digit.

Figure I

Let's begin with the hours' tens digit. There are three possibilities: nothing, 1, and 2. So we need at least two different liquid crystals to distinguish between them. One crystal has only two states, switched on and switched off, and thus can differentiate between only two symbols.

To distinguish nothing from 1, one crystal in the set {3, 6} (see Figure 1) has to be functional. To distinguish 1 from 2, one crystal in the set {1, 4, 5, 7} has to be functional. We then see that if crystals 3 and 5 are functional, we always know what the hours' tens digit is (see Figure 2) and that it is impossible to know this with only one functional crystal.

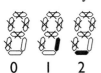

0   1   2

Figure 2: hours' tens digit. One possibility out of eight with two functional crystals.

For the hours' tens digit, we can have at most five nonfunctional liquid crystals.

Let's consider the case of the hours' units digit. There are ten possibilities, all the numbers from 0 to 9.

To distinguish 1 from 7, crystal 1 has to be functional.

To distinguish 6 from 8, crystal 3 has to be functional.

To distinguish 0 from 8, crystal 4 has to be functional.

To distinguish 8 from 9, crystal 5 has to be functional.

But while these four crystals enable us to distinguish between $2 \times 2 \times 2 \times 2 = 16$ theoretical values, they do not enable us to distinguish 2 from 8 and 3 from 9. So we have to add one more functional crystal: crystal 2. With these five functional crystals, we can verify that all numbers can be distinguished from each other (see Figure 3).

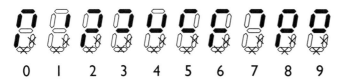

0   1   2   3   4   5   6   7   8   9

Figure 3: hours' units digit. The only possibility with five functional crystals.

For the hours' units digit (and it is the same for the minutes' units digit), we can have at most two nonfunctional liquid crystals.

Let's finally consider the case of the minutes' tens digit. There are six possibilities, the numbers from 0 to 5. To distinguish between these six, we need at least three functional crystals (two functional crystals have at most $2 \times 2 = 4$ possible positions). Crystals 3 and 6, each being used by five of the numbers, are not useful. We then see that crystals 2 and 5 must be functional and that either crystal 1 or crystal 7 must be functional. For the minutes' tens digit, we can have at most four nonfunctional liquid crystals (see Figure 4).

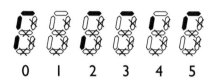

0   1   2   3   4   5

Figure 4: minutes' tens digit. One possibility out of two with three functional crystals.

The maximum number of nonfunctional liquid crystals that enables Nicholas to read the time without ambiguity is $5 + 2 + 4 + 2 = \textbf{13.}$

47. *X* Cannot Live There

Let's first consider the central square of *X*. This square cannot be put on the border squares. With this in mind, only 12 squares remain on which to place the central square of *X* (the white squares in Figure 1).

Any time we color a square black, none of the four adjacent squares can be the central square of *X* (see Figure 2).

We then find that **four** black squares are sufficient (see Figures 3 and 4) to keep *X* out, but that three black squares are not.

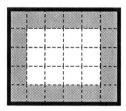

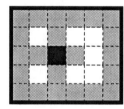

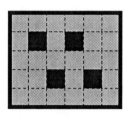

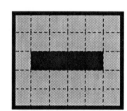

Figure 1   Figure 2   Figure 3   Figure 4

48. A Little Logic

Let us assume that Walter is telling the truth.

- If A were true, B and C would have to be false according to condition 1, so for condition 2 to be true, D would have to be true, but then condition 3 would be false, since A and D would both be true. Thus, A must be false.

- Similar reasoning shows that D cannot be true.

- If B were true, then C and D would have to be false according to condition 2, so condition 3 would be false since both A and D would be false. Thus, B must be false.

- Similar reasoning shows that C cannot be true.

Thus, Walter has lied at least once.

Lydia's statements are consistent. The only true proposition is C: If one of the other propositions is true, say A, then according to conditions 1 and 3, B, C, and D are all false, which contradicts condition 2.

There is only one true proposition: **proposition C.**

49. Master Fibo Unchains Himself

The total number of links is 143. Since $143 = 11 \times 13$, the length of the chains must be 1, 11, or 13.

Let's try the length 13, since we already have a chain of that length. We first separate the chains longer than 13 as shown at right (the opened links are circled).

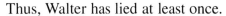

We then obtain, by opening six links, seven chains that are 13 links long plus the existing one. So three chains of 13 links now have to be built with the smaller parts. It can be done as shown, merely by closing links.

It is obvious that we cannot open fewer than six links since we have to cut the longer chains into small parts.

Concerning the length 11, we cannot open fewer than eight links for the same reason.

So the best way to complete the job is to make 11 chains of length 13 with the previous method. It takes 6 link openings and 6 link closings, that is, **6 minutes to complete the job.**

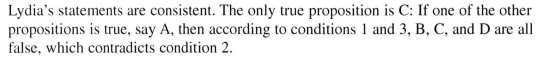

---

50. The Diamond

Since $4 = 3 + 1$ and $5 = 3 + 2$, it will simplify our analysis if we initially treat all numbers "modulo 3"; that is, let "0" represent all multiples of 3, let "1" represent all numbers that are 1 more than a multiple of 3, and let "2" represent all numbers that are 2 more than a multiple of 3. Thus, the difference between two adjacent number representations must be 1 or 2, and no two adjacent number representations can be the same.

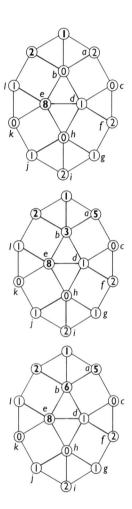

Given the positions of 1, 2, and 8, and remembering that 8 is represented by "2," we complete the diamond in the order b, a and d, c and h, f, g, i, j, k, and l (see figure).

Except for 1, 2, and 8, the numbers split into

multiples of 3: 3, 6, 9, and 12.

multiples of 3 plus 1: 4, 7, 10, and 13.

multiples of 3 plus 2: 5, 11, and 14.

The only possible number that can fill in a is 5 (11 and 14 are too large).

Two numbers can fill in b: 3 and 6.

Let us first use 3. Since only 11 and 14 can fill in f, the only possibility in d is 7 since 4 is too small. So 4 fills in l, 11 fills in f, and 14 fills in i. 12 cannot fill in c nor can it fill in k. So it fills in h.

If 13 fills in j, 10 fills in g, 9 fills in k, and 6 fills in c. This is a possible solution.

If 10 fills in j, 13 fills in g, and 6 and 9 respectively fill in c and k, or fill in k and c. This gives two different solutions.

Let us now assume that 6 fills in b. Then 3 cannot go in c (11 or 14 is in f), nor in h, which is adjacent to d, g, and j (they contain three of the four integers 4, 7, 10, and 13). So 3 fills in k. Since i contains 11 or 14, j necessarily contains 7. So 11 fills in i, 4 fills in l, and 14 fills in f.

As for the remaining numbers, 9 fills in *c,* 12 fills in *h,* 10 fills in *d,* and 13 fills in *g.* This is the fourth solution.

The diamond can be filled in **four different ways,** shown below.

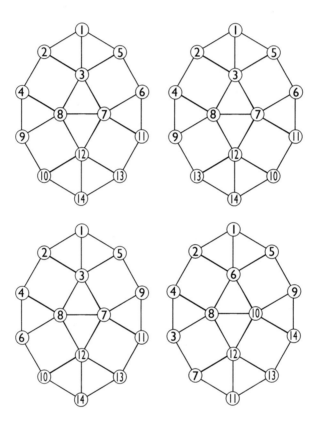

9 781559 534994